THE
PATIENT
IS A
PIGEON

The high cost of blind trust in healthcare

By Dr. Ken Hajek

Published by Dr. Ken Hajek

Sacramento, California

May 2014

ISBN 978-1-312-13826-1

http://straighttalkdental.net/

khajek@strighttalkdental.net

Introduction

When I was a young dentist, I once worked for a small corporate chain as an associate. One dentist did all the exams and an additional four of us did the work he prescribed. It was late winter, gray, and the Central Valley was foggy and cold. Volume was down and Corporate had been talking sternly to the examining dentist about this low "production."

In walked a young woman in her mid-20s. She had only two fillings for all of her years and expected just a cleaning. She went through the normal process and ended up sitting in my dental chair, flustered, with a list of twelve fillings for me to do. Fifteen hundred dollars.

When I checked those problem spots before doing any drilling, I found solid tooth structure in all but two – not decay. The examining dentist had diagnosed tea stains as decay. We identify that kind of decay by probing with a little pick, not visually. This is so basic that it could not have been a mistake on the part of the dentist. I crossed through ten of the planned restorations, did the two tiny ones, and sent her off. Well, she was angry and gave the examining dentist a piece of her mind on the way out. Unaware and trusting, she had been set up to be a pigeon.

I was let go the next day.

Two small fillings served the patient's need. Ten additional, unnecessary fillings were meant to serve the need of the corporation. When you go to the dentist are you sure you need all of that work? Might you be like that young woman, unsuspecting, and ready to bow to the authority of the white coats?

There is a conflict of interest in dentistry. In fact, this conflict exists in most professions. The dental office wants to make money by selling treatment, the more the better. The dental patient wants to buy what is appropriate and necessary, but not more. The dentist's dedication to the patients' interest is supposed to be absolute. Yet dentists are human and the line between serving patients and serving self interest is frequently crossed.

A dentist has great power when he makes his recommendations because the patient does not have the expertise to judge what is needed. Unnecessary treatment can usually be recommended and undertaken without question, for people have faith in the professions. I am here to inform you that such trust is frequently abused. The trusting patient too often becomes the pigeon, mark, sucker, or patsy. Your author is 35 years a dentist, waving my arms and shouting, "Look over here. Something is amiss!"

Please note again: The dentist has great power when he makes his recommendations because the patient is not knowledgeable. Therein lies the solution. Make the patient knowledgeable. The patient can be a skilled shopper in healthcare as they are in much of the rest of the economy.

Of course, we cannot train every person to have the same level of expertise as a dentist. Instead, a second opinion from an experienced dentist who has no conflict of interest can provide the necessary knowledge. People routinely come to my office with confusing and divergent second, third, and fourth opinions because conventional dentists all have financial incentives to sell treatment. The effective second opinion must be divorced from the sale of treatment. That's why at my office, we provide information and advice only. No treatment, no conflict.

Overtreatment is not confined to dentistry; it is common throughout the healthcare field because professionals everywhere are human. That means they respond to incentives, regulations and financial pressures, even when their purest intent is to serve patients. Overtreatment results not only in patients receiving services they do not need, but also in hugely inflated medical care costs.

Empowering individuals to be careful shoppers – arming them so they can recognize overtreatment and avoid it – can control costs and protect patients as no government regulation or bureaucrat can. With empowered consumers, you get motivated micromanagement of each individual case to serve the patient rather than the provider, the insurer, or the bureaucrat. You eliminate unnecessary treatment, a major contributor to cost. And you leave the provider's desire to offer and deliver service undiminished by excessive regulation, so care is available.

The definitive healthcare solution lies with the individual, not government mandates and red tape. Read on to see how dentistry works behind the scenes and draw your own conclusions...

Table of Contents

1. THE BUSINESS OF DENTISTRY 1

2. THE BUSINESS OF INSURANCE 15

3. THE PATIENT 21

4. THE DOCTOR.. 23

5. WHY IT ALL GOES WRONG 27

6. THE CURE.. 29

7. STRAIGHT TALK DENTAL 33

8. A FINAL WORD 35

The Patient is a Pigeon

1. The Business of Dentistry

One dentist had a practice in the Sacramento area that brought in $150,000 a year. That may sound like a lot, but it is very low for a dental business. The cost of rent, staff, equipment, education loans and much more likely consumed it all, with zero salary for himself. Then he apparently made a decision to make his business successful. A few years later, he was taking in $750,000 a year, a very respectable figure.

However, his ambition put the business of dentistry ahead of his patients' needs. His downfall was related in a story in the Sacramento Bee titled "Dentist the Menace." The case is still in court, but it is alleged that he did fillings, crowns, root canals and other treatment that was unnecessary, particularly when the patients had generous insurance plans. There were enough complaints after several years of operation at that high level that the Dental Board pulled his license and he was indicted.

This dentist is but the tip of the iceberg. Dentistry is a business, and many dentists focus on business when the patient should be their sole concern.

The Legal Structure

There is long-standing law on the books that only dentists can own dental offices. The dentist is supposed to be the one with ethics to resist an environment filled with business incentives. Other businessmen or investor-owners might push for profit at the expense of the patient, so the law restricted ownership.

More recently, politicians made an exception to this law, opening the door to HMO-type organizations. These can have owners and investors that need not be dentists. In a small practice the dentist with his ethics is in control. In an HMO practice, the front-line dentist is demoted to a third-tier employee in a sales-oriented culture. This puts him under great pressure to sell treatment.

Today, dental HMOs in the form of corporate dental office chains dot the landscape. Their business-oriented model has been financially successful and they are said to deliver one-fourth of the dental care in the nation.

The HMO structure has had effects well beyond its market-share. Impressionable dentists just out of school often work in a chain office to get a start. When they eventually move out on their own, they may take those business practices and that business-oriented attitude into their new private practices. An overdeveloped business orientation is the new normal for dentists within an HMO structure, for dentists who used to be in one, and for dentists copying that financially successful model.

The Philosophical Split

My personal experience and observations lead me to believe that 50 percent of the people in the profession are traditional patient-oriented dentists. That half is generally aware of the practices of the other, business-oriented half, and there is a tension between the two.

At a social event some time ago, I met the wife of a Northern California dentist. The woman's husband was approaching retirement and was considering selling his practice. A younger dentist across town wanted to buy the practice.

However, the philosophical split in the profession was causing the older dentist to hesitate. His dental hygienist daughter had worked for the younger dentist for a time. She told her father that the younger dentist was what she called a "seller." She meant he was a business-oriented dentist who pushed sales to benefit his business. The old-school dentist was in the other camp, patient-oriented and protective of his people. Although that sale would have been easy and profitable, the older dentist decided that he would forego the opportunity and not sell to this younger dentist.

His wife was very supportive of my effort to help patients with unbiased advice, as other dentists and hygienists have been. However, the economic forces that move a dentist from our camp over to what I call "The Dark Side" of the profession are powerful.

Money Pressure

As indicated above, dentists come in two flavors: the small, private practice owner-operator and the dentist-employee. Both can be influenced by the business of dentistry and a constant pressure for income.

The owner-operator has to cover his costs every month, and these are substantial. Staff and rent are the biggest, but there are many others. A dentist's investment in seven or eight years of higher education means student loans to repay. If the dentist buys a practice he must also pay back a purchase loan that is typically about half a million dollars. Add in the normal expenses of life – car, house, kids, insurance, food, fuel, and so on – and you can imagine the stress and financial pressure on the dentist. He needs not only many patients but also enough work to do on those patients every month to make it balance. There is no guarantee that those patients will come through the door, and sometimes they do not.

This economic stress exists alongside the stress of working around peoples' nerve endings in a confined area under time pressure. The stress can be severe, and dentists have long had the highest suicide rate of any profession.

So private practitioners are one flavor. The employee-dentist, the other flavor, is also subject to economic pressure. Dentist-employees are rated by Corporate on how many dollars each has "produced." Additional stats are kept on other aspects: Dollars-per-appointment and percentage of treatment plans "sold" are typical. The dentist's financial performance is thoroughly analyzed. Low numbers put the dentist's job at risk and, as dentists are usually contracted employees, there is no job security.

How Offices Make More Money (at the Patient's Expense)

Like other businesses, dental offices sometimes call in consultants for advice on how to make more money. An office engaged one such consultant while I worked there as an associate. His $60,000 fee included lectures, staff training, modified front desk practices, and so on over a month or two.

Much of the training was about sales. We were taught that "the patient has the money for their dental work. They just spend it in other places." We were taught how to advance the prospects for a "sale" by letting the patient "overhear" part of the sales pitch discussed by other staff. The "closer" was taught to "echo" the words of the doctor to give them greater weight. Nodding and smiling were encouraged. Use fear of tooth loss or heart problems (there is an established link) to help sell procedures. And so on. Manipulation of the patient, not merit of the necessary dental work.

Then he left, having imparted his aggressive business attitude, a few tricks, and little else.

What follows are a number of technical and procedural methods used in business-oriented practices.

1. Changing Standards

In dental school, the standard is perfection. When dentists get out into the work-a-day world, they perform to a high standard but not to that of dental-school perfection. So when a dentist's business is short of work, one solution is for the dentist to move his personal standards up a few notches closer to dental-school perfection. The following are examples:

4

- The slight irregularity in the crown margin that wouldn't trouble a busy dentist can become a reason to re-do the crown for $1,000.
- When probing the gums to decide between a regular cleaning and a deep cleaning, just be a little more critical. The decision to do a deep cleaning can add $1,000 to production.
- Aging fillings that might have another decade of service in them are showing a few signs of wear? They suddenly must be replaced.
- Or after deciding to replace that filling, by being hyper-safe regarding what can be a very low risk of fracture, a dentist can sell a crown instead for seven-times the dollar volume.

2. Prevention by Restoration

Dentists usually think of prevention as toothbrush, floss, and instruction toward the prevention of decay and gum disease. The purpose is to avoid the need for restoration. "Prevention by restoration" turns such common-sense on its head.

Prevention by restoration was common in what we used to call DentiCal mills. These were offices that served the state dental program for the poor in California. Compensation from the state declined steadily over time. Yet the DentiCal offices had to try to make it work, given the reductions.

One of the ways was prevention by restoration. One makes the cynical assumption that the vulnerable areas between the teeth are ultimately going to develop decay. Instead of doing them one at a time as they become decayed and incurring higher costs, a dentist fills all of the surfaces now that *might* decay in the future. This can triple the dollar volume per unit of time and, in the face of declining government funding, keep the office in business. The patient, however, is ill-served.

3. The Upsell

A patient already needs a crown. Insurance will cover the cost of an ordinary crown but the fee is relatively low. So the upsell pitch is that it would be better to use a "higher-quality" crown. The "higher quality" is a change of the supporting metal to gold. It is true that there is a slight color advantage in some situations, but these recommendations are not limited to those applications. There is an additional out-of-pocket fee and it can add 20 percent to the price of a crown.

4. Add-ons

Perhaps you've taken your car to an auto shop for an oil change. They always find something else, don't they? "Your reservoirs are down," or something "needs replacement." How about the car dealer, having sold a car, who pushes a costly warranty? Add-ons like these can add significant dollar volume to the bottom line of the seller.

Add-ons exist in dentistry, too. Some offices routinely recommend additional procedures when they recommend a deep cleaning, and sell three procedures as a linked package instead of one. Laser cautery and antibiotic therapy, linked to deep cleaning, can add $1,000 to the bill but are of questionable long-term benefit.

Bone grafts can be another add-on. The conventional practice is to use bone grafts selectively in specific situations. Some offices advocate a bone graft procedure for *every* extraction. The procedure requires only a few minutes and can add up to $500 to the bill.

When corporate clinics find "profit centers" like bone grafts, laser cautery, or antibiotic therapy, they pointedly suggest that their employee-dentists push those procedures more aggressively.

5. *X-rays*

X-ray machines have come a long way since I first became a dentist. Films have improved, exposure times are lower, and shielding is more complete. But the frequency with which a dentist should take x-rays has not changed. A full series every seven to ten years and a few checkup x-rays annually are quite adequate.

However some offices use x-rays as a profit center. They take x-rays every checkup visit. X-rays are so common that this can help generate more business income.

It can be said that more frequent x-rays provide better documentation for legal defense. In addition, frequent x-rays compensate for the poor quality of those taken by undertrained staff. However, income is the primary motivation and one should limit patient x-ray exposure to what is truly necessary.

6. *X-ray Interpretation*

One can improve treatment "sales" with liberal interpretation of x-rays, too. For example:

- A dark shadow at the end of a root can indicate the need for a root canal – or it can be a healthy area of the skeleton that is just thin.
- A dark shadow on a tooth can be caused by decay – or it can be caused by the natural shape of the tooth.

7. *Timing of Work*

For patients, there is very little positive about a trip to the dentist. Although nothing hurts, they may be told that something is wrong. They then must devote time, money, inconvenience, and perhaps discomfort to this previously unknown issue. Given this, many people have to work up the courage to go, and when they're in the chair they tell us they hate to be there.

If you do have pain, it's a different story. Dental pain can really get your attention and ruin your day. So when pain brings you to the dental chair, you are already motivated to buy. And dentists are happy to sell. But the business-aggressive ones will try to push everything they can while the patient is motivated, because they might not come back once the pain diminishes.

For example, it's very common for a person to come in with the pain of a toothache when the nerve of a tooth is infected. We normally fix these with a root canal, but patient-oriented offices will quell the infection, reduce the pain and schedule the root canal a week later. In contrast, business-oriented offices will sell the root canal, tooth buildup, and crown on the spot and do the work that same day.

Unfortunately, infections can negate the effect of anesthetics. Doing a root canal on a tooth that won't get numb can be torture. It is not uncommon to hear a patient in agony in the next room when a business-oriented dentist has that happen and proceeds anyway.

Sometimes there is a question about exactly which tooth is causing pain. It is rare for more than one tooth to be causing a problem at one time, but it can be difficult to identify exactly which one it is.

Business-oriented offices will sometimes do root canals on every tooth in the area to be sure to get a problem one. That practice allows them to proceed with work immediately, be sure of solving the problem, and put higher "production" numbers on the board. In contrast, patient-oriented offices will wait a week and undertake diagnostic tests to determine which one tooth needs that root canal.

The push for immediate work also can be short-sighted. Business-oriented offices will often sell $2,000 of work for one tooth with a root canal, buildup, and crown because the patient is focused on pain in that tooth. In the push for "production," little attention is given to the general state of the rest of the patient's teeth or their financial means. All too often the patient's budget is expended to repair only one tooth, they don't return and the rest of the teeth continue to deteriorate. Patient-oriented offices evaluate the whole mouth. The $2,000 may be better applied in repair of half-a-dozen lesser decay spots.

8. Dentistry by the Book

"Policy", or doing dental work by the book, can justify some charges when common sense would go another direction.

One young nineteen-year-old male ended up in my corporate-office chair one busy day. I was assigned to do a deep cleaning based on another dentist's diagnosis.

Now, one determines that a deep cleaning is needed by putting a measuring probe alongside the tooth to see how far down the gums are attached. A normal reading is three millimeters. Five millimeters is deep. The examining dentist had measured this young fellow's depths and prescribed the deep cleaning.

By the book, this young fellow needed that $1,000 of work because the depths qualified. However, when I looked at his situation I found no deterioration. Bone loss would have been very unusual for someone at his age anyway. The measurements were five millimeters because he did not brush his teeth regularly and his gums were swollen and puffed up. What he needed was not a $1,000 cleaning, but a $2.50 toothbrush.

I gave him the toothbrush and some instruction and sent him away without the deep cleaning. Ten days later, his gums were normal and he had a regular cleaning that cost less than $100. Management was displeased.

9. Corporate Practices

Corporate chains have made many adaptations to improve their business net. Few, if any, are patient-focused.

- Office managers used to be dentists. Corporations decided they could cut that cost by giving those management duties to a dental assistant instead. This move saves on salary but further elevates the business aspects above patient-related ones.

- There is usually a specialist "closer" to undertake the financial arrangements, just like with car sales. It goes like this. You see the doctor for the exam, but he goes away while you wait. After a time, the closer comes in with the proposed treatment plan, the costs and a contract. "The doctor says you need x, y, and z. How would you like to pay?" Or "Your portion after insurance is $$. How would you like to pay?" And "we have payment plans." If you have questions, they provide generic explanations and occasionally an outright lie, but their primary goal is to close the sale. Closers typically receive a bonus for high sales numbers.

- Dentists with high "production" earn bonuses, too. High production is less a matter of how hard you work than of how aggressively you diagnose. Thus, a dentist has a direct self-interest in "finding" lots of work on each patient.

Some corporate offices have patients see whichever dentist is available at the given time to better keep the dentists busy. This means that you don't get to see the same dentist on different visits and there is little continuity in the handling of your case because dentists have disparate opinions.

In one such office, a lady was brought to me to have her teeth cleaned and we had an introductory conversation. She had seen three or four different dentists in her recent appointments and each wanted to do different things. In most cases, the list was extensive.

After she explained all of this, she looked up from the chair with a lost expression on her face and asked very sincerely, "Do I really need all that work?" So I did my own brief exam. No, she didn't need all of the work listed. I told her so, but sotto voce because conservative diagnosis – especially reducing already diagnosed work – was frowned upon by management and Corporate.

Corporate offices also want to keep the dentist very busy. A common practice is to have several cases going at once in separate rooms. This tends to leave patients unattended for extended periods while in treatment.

I once worked in a corporate office that lined up more patients than usual. We worked in a converted bank building and there were many rooms. Staff kept the rooms filled so we three dentists could move from room to room, but with so many patients they could not be closely attended.

Operations were downstairs and the staff lunchroom was upstairs. It was a lazy summertime afternoon and I had just finished my late lunch upstairs. I walked down the stairs toward the rest of my afternoon schedule. As I went through the door into the lobby area and the door closed behind me, I suddenly heard a strained voice: "There's a dentist!"

I looked up to see fifteen or twenty people looking at me, including a father holding his rag-doll, unconscious son upright a few feet away. One of the other dentists had parked this sixteen year-old in a chair, applied local anesthetic, and moved on while it took effect. This is customary practice. The dentist was now off on break and the boy had been unattended.

Fortunately, the father had come to keep his fair-haired son company. At some point he had been unable to rouse him.

He then picked him up and carried him to the lobby to seek help.

The assistants were wide-eyed. Emergencies are very rare in general dentistry, and this was a shock and surprise. With my return from lunch, I was the only one on the floor, so everyone was focused on me.

I motioned to the floor and went down on my knees. I took a second to compose myself while they put the boy in front of me, his legs akimbo. His pulse at the neck told me his heart was really racing, but he was pale as a ghost. Our local anesthetics can do that, because some contain adrenalin, but it was probably made worse as the father clasped his arms around the boy's chest to carry him to the lobby. That would have restricted his breathing.

The boy appeared to be breathing and his heart was working overtime, so he didn't need CPR. We'll get blood to his head by elevating his feet, I thought. I glanced up for assistance but everyone seemed frozen, watching. So I reached over and brought his legs up. It took two tries, but I got them to stay in position. I had moved toward his head again to recheck his vital signs when I saw his eyelids flutter and I knew we were OK. What a relief! As he opened his eyes, I sat back and said, "Welcome back; you fainted."

No harm was done, but patient-oriented offices keep better watch on their patients.

A different corporate characteristic showed itself when a provider organization that I worked for took on a new contract. Corporate wanted to grow the number of patients served. They took over a capitation plan from another contractor and added thousands of patients to their roster. Capitation plans pay a small monthly fee per covered person whether they come in or not, but then there is no charge for the enrolled person when they need care. Providers make money because not everyone comes in.

However, in this case management took on the patients without expanding capacity. We suddenly had hundreds of people clamoring to be seen. The front desk booked as many as they could, and we dentists ended up trying to see too many patients to do anything positive. A normal workday is ten to fifteen patients. In this case they booked over fifty patients a day and seemed to expect us to make it work. With a patient every ten minutes, one can achieve little. There was lots of prescription writing, because that is quick, but we were still spinning our wheels.

One could state that these insured patients had dental coverage and service, but our care-delivery was so overloaded that in fact they did not.

10. Color Coding

The business of dentistry requires money. It is possible to have lots of patients with lots of work and still have low income. That way lays business failure. It can happen with poor compensation schedules. So offices pay attention to the nature of each person's means of payment and their insurance coverage.

Business-oriented offices pay particularly close attention. It was common to have front-desk corporate-office assistants hurry to the back, excited to tell the waiting dentists that the next exam patient had a good plumbers' union plan or was paying cash. Management would take special note of that kind of patient because good plans or cash brought in a disproportionate part the day's income. It was expected that you would diagnose lots of work on those patients. If you did not, management would express disappointment and displeasure. Corporate executives might even call later in the day to ask the office manager about such a case. People with good dental insurance and income from a job are particular targets for business-oriented offices.

Corporate offices hungry for more patients – and most are – tend to accept low-compensation plans. Government plans are often that type, for politicians will vote for benefits but provide only inadequate funding. The corporations that accept low-compensation plans develop policies to adapt.

I once worked in a large corporate clinic that accepted a county plan for the poor. Corporate made it work by color-coding the charts to prioritize each patient. Green was cash or excellent insurance, other colors were intermediate plans, and the government plans were red or yellow. The government compensation was low. We were instructed to use the red or yellow charts as filler for otherwise idle time. If emergency work was not needed for these patients, we were to do the lowest cost procedure first, but we were limited to only one procedure per month per person. We saw a great deal of need and, because of these restrictions, were unable to address it properly. It was troubling.

Worse yet, waiting times frequently went hours, even for previously scheduled appointments, because more advantageously colored charts were seen first. Many times I heard harsh words from families on that plan after they had waited several hours with young children.

Color coding of charts also created a serious game among dentists. A dentist with good-paying charts can make his quota while a dentist with predominantly poor-paying charts must struggle. The game was to position yourself to be selectively assigned the "good" charts so as to keep your production numbers up. In offices where charts were assigned, "good" charts were more likely to go to dentists willing to aggressively diagnose problems that required profit-making treatments.

2. The Business of Insurance

Dentists get only occasional glimpses of other dentists' work. Dental assistants see all of a dentist's practices, step-by-step, as they do it. One day in conversation, my dental assistant told me about one of her previous employers...

This dentist accepted some very low-fee insurance plans as a "preferred provider." Some of those insurance plans paid nothing for regular cleanings and only one-fifth of a normal fee for a deep cleaning. The cleaning-oriented part of an exam is to examine a patient's gums, measure depths at six places around every tooth, and call out those millimeter readings to the assistant for her to record in the chart. Two and three millimeter readings are normal and warrant a regular cleaning procedure. If there are many five millimeter readings, one recommends a deep cleaning.

So when this dentist saw patients for those exams he would probe three places around one molar on the lower left, three places around one molar on the lower right, then turn to the assistant and tell her to record five or six millimeter readings around all of the back teeth. That documentation would then justify a deep cleaning.

A bad dentist? Perhaps, but how about a bad insurance company? Insurance companies restrict patient choice to be able to "sell" bodies to dental offices most desperate for them. Those insurance plans leave a dental office with three choices: Do not accept the insurance and have your business fail for lack of patients. Accept the insurance and work at those below-cost fees, lose money, and have your business fail for lack of money. Or find ways to game the system, as the dentist above did.

The insurance companies serve themselves above all, and those self-serving practices have created business models that take advantage of the patient.

The Nature of Insurers

The number one task of insurers is not patient well-being. It is to make money. The money they make ultimately comes from the patient, but its circuitous route masks that fact. If an employer writes a check to the insurance company, that is compensation for work time just as much as one's paycheck. However because it takes this tax-law incentivized route (blame the politicians), people don't look at it as "their" money.

This compromises one of the primary motivations to be a smart shopper, and makes life much easier for the insurer and provider. Their message to the consumer is, "We'll take care of you." The unspoken follow-up should be "...in ways that serve our income."

You must follow the money to understand the business of insurance, for insurers are green-eyeshade guys with very sharp pencils. They set up their models and projections and follow them closely. Although priced and represented differently, their money is a "cut" of the money that passes through their hands. Sell more policies, cover more people, handle more money, and the insurer makes more money.

2The insurers' cost controls extend only as far as their money-making interests and are relatively low-cost in themselves. Companies use x-ray reviews, preauthorizations, data mining, and chart reviews and are able to control some costs, but they do not protect the patient and a lot of unnecessary treatment goes through their screens. They protect their "cut" of the money handled by making sure costs fit their projections. They also want to project a cost-control image for the purpose of marketing new policies. Major cost reductions are not sought after, as any substantial reduction in claims would ultimately cut insurer income.

I had a conversation with a retired insurance CEO some years back. He had semi-retired to golf and a small suburban insurance business with his daughter. He considered dental insurance a no-brainer and a backwater compared to medical insurance because the financial risk was so contained. Average dental claims run only a few hundred dollars per person per year and there's an annual cap. He declared that dental insurance runs very true to their models and garners little attention. But that was his orientation, financial risk and money management. The patient never came up.

An insurer has a business or a banker's orientation. That is their job and they make money doing it. Each patient needs to understand that they are a number on a chart; not an individual, but part of a group.

Were insurers interested in dental patient well-being, we would not be spending over $80 billion annually on dental work today, and the insurer's piece of the pie would be smaller. We have known for 50 years how to prevent tooth decay and gum disease; still the bulk of the money today goes for those continuing problems.

Prevention instruction, if done properly, can take 15 minutes of chair time. Many people put great effort into their homecare, but still have decay or gum problems because there are flaws in their technique or understanding.

Some think a hard toothbrush is desirable. That's a problem because the bristles do not flex to get into the recesses at the gum line and between the teeth where the bacteria are otherwise undisturbed. Some brush vigorously back to front. That doesn't allow time enough for the bristles to hit more than the high points and once again the recesses are left undisturbed.

Soft bristles and a short, circular motion on both gums and teeth are what I call for, both in the morning after breakfast and at night before bed. Those who don't clean before sleeping have more trouble because food residue feeds the bacteria through the night, compared to a short time during the day. One can mimic that long exposure time by frequent snacking and create the same problems, too. Sip a soda or coffee with sugar through the day, have a candy habit (including breath mints), or indulge often in anything with sugar, and we will see you at the office much more frequently.

Flossing is another area for better instruction. When I finish instructing, many 50- and 60-year-old patients tell me that they've never been told how to floss properly despite many years of cleanings. Movie scenes that show flossing with hands held far apart drive us dentists crazy because the technique is poor.

One should choke up on the floss and not pull it excessively tight or straight as you wipe the tooth surfaces free of plaque. The purpose of floss is to wipe clean the surfaces your toothbrush won't reach, not to remove fiber. It is of note that a tooth has the shape of a cylinder. If one keeps the floss straight instead of wrapping around the curvature of the cylinder, one cleans only a skinny line on the surface instead of cleaning the whole thing. If you pull the floss in and out you clean only a horizontal skinny line. We want you to wipe the whole surface clean.

It is common for gums to be tender or to bleed, but what is common is not healthy. That's literally a red flag that your home care is not doing the job or you need a cleaning at the office. Ten days of brushing and flossing properly should make the bleeding go away. If your technique is correct, you can even miss flossing once in a while (we recommend once daily at night) and be just fine.

Most people now brush their teeth and many floss, but everyone seems to make their own mistakes in technique or habit. Decay bacteria are relentless and take advantage. Video instruction or mass instruction techniques are nowhere near as effective as a one-on-one session, and one such visit can prevent a lifetime of decay.

But back to the insurers and their effect on prevention. Superficially the insurers appear to pay attention to prevention and maintenance. Some will offer policies that provide free or very-low cost cleanings, with the idea that more cleanings will prevent problems. It is subtle but actually deceptive, and benefits the insurer.

Cleanings at the dentist do not provide good oral health; good home care does. Good home care comes from prevention instruction. Prevention instruction is not a separate item on a contracted fee schedule, but is supposed to be done with a cleaning and compensated within that fee. By reducing the fee or making it zero, the insurers effectively pressure the dentist to minimize time spent on it. It also puts the onus on the dentist if it is poorly done or not done at all, so insurers can put their hands up, Bart Simpson-like, declaring "we didn't do it." This behind-the-scenes economic disincentive effectively reduces prevention and keeps the treatment dollars flowing.

In one corporate chain I was instructed: "At each cleaning, say something brief about tooth brushing, then document in the chart that OHI [oral hygiene instruction] was done." That creates the paper trail so the appropriate box can be checked on an insurance audit and you can get right into the hands-on cleaning part that actually justifies any fee. Insurer manipulation and provider response together set patients up so they return with new work to be done every few years.

Another thing insurers do is restrict patient choice. We do not have a free market for care because the insurers have Balkanized it with their "networks" of providers. They effectively limit who you can see for treatment. Titled "Preferred Providers," they are actually networks of the lowest bidders. And you get what you pay for. As described earlier, providers take note of the payment plan and respond variously by cutting corners, tapping the patient's pocket directly, or gaming the system.

Insurance companies are a big business. Dentistry is but a collection of small businesses. It is an imbalance that has allowed the insurance industry to shape rules and practices to their purposes, as avid sellers seeking profit. Of course there is nothing wrong with seeking profit, for that is necessary to business. Self interest and the search for profit are what gives vitality to our system.

The problem lies not with the insurers, but with a structure that has no effective counterparty in the buyer. Lacking such balance, insurers have been able to do disservice to patients with the restriction of patient choice, creation of an exploitative business model, and the sly suppression of prevention. If we re-empower patients as the ultimate buyers and get politicians to reshape the insurer rules, we can establish a balance that provides good service to the patient and keeps the sellers in check.

3. The Patient

Charles is in his mid-70s and tries to take good care of himself, teeth, gums and all. He gets a dental checkup every six months, regular as clockwork. So after the cleaning at one checkup, the dentist did his exam and seemed to find nothing, as had been Charles' history, until the very end when he lingered on one crown. "It needs to be replaced," he said. "There's decay there."

Charles said okay and was ready to schedule an appointment when the dentist added that there would be an out-of-pocket extra charge to make the new crown fit with his existing situation. Charles almost went ahead anyway; we are conditioned to trust what the doctor says, after all. But an extra $75? He came to see me for a second opinion.

I checked the tooth and found nothing wrong, though Charles didn't want me to take an x-ray that visit. A few weeks passed and Charles called again. He wanted his money back. He had gone to a health fair where a dentist was taking free Panorex x-rays. As the doctor examined his free x-ray, Charles casually asked whether that crown in question needed to be replaced. The doctor looked at the x-ray and told him yes. So Charles called to chew me out. We talked and I offered to double check it.

He came to the office and I looked at the tooth again. This time I took a cavity-check type of x-ray too. Everything was normal. There was no decay. The health fair doctor's Panorex x-ray is a scan of the whole mouth, normally used for surgical procedure and orthodontia, not to diagnose decay. Bad information from two of three doctors? What's a patient to do?

Americans are smart shoppers in most of the economy, but when it comes to being a patient, that skill usually isn't applied. Three things get in the way: the Discipline, Deference and Disinterest.

"The Discipline" refers to professional dental knowledge and its complexity. There is a lot to know and the layman can't hope to master it. The knowledge, experience and judgment necessary to be a smart shopper reside exclusively in a dentist.

Deference. Patients respect and trust those in the professions. That has become less true with the advent of the Internet and easier ways for people to research their options or tap into other people's experiences. Nonetheless, most patients continue to believe whatever the professional in the white coat tells them.

Disinterest. Dentistry is a small part of our lives and we have bigger things to do with our time than pay close attention to it. It is infrequent, cost is not a big concern because many people have insurance, and we're usually not in pain. So we'd rather not think about it.

Yet as a cautious shopper, how far do you drive to save 20 cents on a gallon of gas? Does 20 cents or 50 cents per pound of fruit make a difference to you? How far would you go to save $20 on an item? Every day, people work through all the advertising, images, marketing and blather that the sellers throw at them and they still manage to make good purchasing decisions for products and simple services. Yet the same person will write out a $2,000 check to the dentist rather casually, shopping skills absent.

4. The Doctor

I was a young dentist in private practice in a mid-sized Valley town. I met a dentist a few years my senior in town. He was a very sincere fellow, earnest in his specialty practice that dealt with people's gum conditions. He had an attractive wife and two young kids, a suburban house in a nice neighborhood, and a nice life.

He was ambitious, as many dentists are. You must be to become a dentist, for the selection process had ten or more applications for each dental school slot in my day and it's worse now. This dentist was not content with the success of his practice. He sought professional stature.

There is a pecking order in healthcare, with surgeons and medical specialists at the top, and physicians and others in some unofficial descending order. Dentists perceive themselves to be lower-ranking but within that family. Physicians think of them as distant, hardly related cousins. Maybe we try harder for that.

In any case, many dentists are actually frustrated would-be doctors. In the time frame of this incident with this Valley dentist, there was a big push for our profession to assume more doctor-like duties. Some dental schools even changed the dentists' degrees from Doctor of Dental Surgery (DDS) to Doctor of Medical Dentistry (DMD). Perhaps it's a tiny step closer to medicine in some people's minds.

In any case, we dentists were newly tasked with taking a patient's blood pressure, screening for head and neck cancer, and other things.

This periodontist had risen relatively high within dentistry by becoming a specialist, but he did not seem satisfied. He wanted to be the best in his specialty as well, and was an early-adopter of the newest trends, including the new screening practices.

Accepted cancer screening includes feeling for lymph nodes in the head and neck. Lymph nodes are normally small, but if they're enlarged it can be an indicator of infection or cancer, so a dentist or doctor has to feel around. Palpation – to examine part of the body with hands and fingers – of head and neck muscles was also encouraged, as tender muscles can indicate a jaw dysfunction called TMJ syndrome.

This dentist sought to push the boundaries to be on the cutting edge, and it is my suspicion that his perception slipped. There are lymph nodes in the armpit area that he might have checked, and then he went a step too far. Screening for breast cancer has been a medical focus for a long time. Were he a doctor-doctor, it would have been routine, but he was a dentist-doctor working below the neck. Definitely a no-go area.

He was charged, there was a big write-up in the paper (sex sells) and, though I don't know the legal outcome, he moved away.

Dentists are generally good people, but a dentist is human. The economic and societal environments affect us, and the isolation, power, and economic pressures of our profession can make one's perceptions slip. Isolation, because the dentist usually does his work alone. Power, because he alone knows his complex discipline and speaks its language – the patient does not. And we've already described the economic pressures.

If your perceptions slip, then "restoration for prevention," "more treatment is better care," and a business orientation can seem reasonable. This is especially true as the financial success of the HMO model has institutionalized that business orientation.

Slipped perception is common to all of the professions. Many dentists, doctors, lawyers, and politicians think they are great.

I listened to a radio interview in which a doctor said that many physicians saw innovation in electronic monitoring of patients as a threat to their "authority." Authority is defined as the "right to command: the right or power to enforce rules or give orders." I personally don't see where doctors have any such right regarding patients. But that perspective is entrenched.

Look at the phrasing that one needs to be "released " from a hospital. Doctors as commanders and hospitals as prisons? Is inflated self-importance not a slipped perception?

5. Why It All Goes Wrong

I recently moved, and ended up far away from my old auto mechanic. The guy was a classic grease monkey. He owned his own shop and loved what he did. His work was cars. His hobby was cars. He was always a little disheveled, working in the shop bays himself, but he looked out for you. If there were another 5,000 miles in a tire, he'd say so and let you decide. If he could cut the cost with a rebuilt part, and he felt it would be reliable, he'd sell you that lower-priced item. Trustworthy.

So it became time for an oil change in my new location and I ended up at a local franchise shop. The manager didn't get his hands dirty. The paperwork was fast and flawless. The oil change wasn't cheap in itself, and then the manager came into the waiting room. "We found something."

He wanted to sell me a new engine belt as the old one had some minor, very hard-to-discern cracks from age. I declined, but there is the difference. One guy watches out for you and another tries to sneak an extra sale off of you.

That effort to sneak an extra sale off of you is an expression of human nature. Literally. It is in the <u>nature</u> of humans to serve self and family first. The mechanic seeking the extra sale valued his business gain over selfless service to the customer.

Dentistry is like that. Selfless service is the concept that goes wrong. While true for perhaps half of the profession, the other half values that self-interested "business orientation" over selfless service to the patient.

Now, a business orientation works fine in the rest of the economy. Avid sellers are out plying their products and services, using every trick in the book. Their eagerness to sell makes things readily available and the seller responsive. Consumers shop for price, quality and service every day, and they are skilled at it. So there exists a balance: cautious consumers are pitted against avid sellers.

Professional services are different. Humans staffing the professions are supposed to serve others as the priority. Human genetics, however, program us to serve self and family. Business orientation with dentists and doctors or self-interest with lawyers and politicians is just Mother Nature showing through. Those relationships lack balance and the avid sellers thrive in the face of a passive consumer, a pigeon.

The consumer is made more passive yet through trust in the concept of selfless professions. Trust is defined as "reliance: confidence in a reliance on good qualities, especially fairness, truth, honor, or ability." "Reliance." Did you ever "rely" on or depend on someone, only to be disappointed? Professionals are human, too. Blind trust or reliance can be misplaced and the consumer will never know.

6. The Cure

We have been moving responsibilities away from the individual toward insurance groups for years, and ultimately toward government management with the Affordable Care Act. In dentistry, we have gone from a one-on-one relationship with the dentist, to being part of a limited-choice insurance group, toward being a government statistic. Each move in that direction diminishes the individual and his or her needs and concerns. To paraphrase a famous quotation: One incident is a tragedy, a million is a statistic.

Government oversight adds a layer of self-interested politicians and bureaucrats to the mix – and how often do those elites manage efficiently, conserve money or reduce costs? It is extremely rare. Besides which the task would be herculean. In dentistry alone a professional sees ten to twenty patients per day, and there are lots of dentists.

Regulatory mechanisms are slow, legalistic and after-the-fact. In fact, government actions taken at the behest of sellers, have created some of the problems in the first place. Government is not a practical solution, for in that direction lays ever-increasing dysfunction. Advisory practices – my recommended cure – would move in the other direction, toward patient control.

The advisory practice would be a positive and minimalist cure; jiu-jitsu rather than sumo. It would be private-sector and directly address the fundamental problem: that the sellers have the run of the place and the skilled shopper that keeps sellers in check elsewhere in the economy is absent here. It has been incremental, but the sellers' advantage has steadily expanded healthcare's "take" to where it is now, double that of other developed countries as a share of GDP. Our obesity epidemic extends to our healthcare sector – fat and definitely not healthy for the rest of us.

Negative regulation of the sellers would be coercive, fight a tide of human self interest and be very complex. The positive approach is to bring patient activity up rather than push seller activity down. What the patient is lacking is technical advice. Patients cannot become suitably knowledgeable themselves, but they can hire that expertise. Unbiased, independent second opinions can activate the shopper within and break the unquestioned power that professionals have over the layman.

The new advisory offices would provide exams, x-rays and advice, including prevention instruction. These offices would strictly NOT offer treatment, for a second opinion from an office that also wants to sell treatment remains suspect because of conflict of interest. Telephone support alone would be inadequate. Actual office visits are necessary because patient hearsay over the telephone, even with x-rays, allows misrepresentations to persist. A consulting dentist needs see the situation directly to make his own appraisal.

Advisory offices fill the bill for cost control: it is accomplished on a case-by-case basis by the individual most involved; there is no rationing of care; the patient is empowered; and the provider's desire to offer and deliver service goes undiminished.

Advisory offices will breach the Wizard-of-Oz curtain surrounding dental professionals and lessen deference and disinterest as people come to understand the extent of unnecessary treatment and unnecessary cost.

Advisory offices provide the information necessary for the patient to fill the role of the cautious shopper, but another change is needed so that shopper can shop freely. Insurance companies severely restrict choices for dental and medical treatment. The necessary change would be to free that market. Allow the insured to shop freely among treatment providers without restriction or penalty. Auto insurance allows car owners to select any provider for repairs. Healthcare insurance should too.

The last tweak to the system should be to move prevention education away from treatment offices where it fares poorly and into the advisory offices. Once in a lifetime, one-on-one individualized instruction is necessary to be truly effective. It should have a separate fee and be adequately compensated, for prevention is health.

These relatively simple measures – power to the patient, freedom of choice, and wellness instruction – can ultimately reduce expenditures for general dentistry by half while providing better service.

7. Straight Talk Dental

My solution comes not just from observation and analysis, but from experience. I started offering dental advisory services of the type referred to above in a prototype office in 2012. We called the operation Second Opinion Dental (later switching to Straight Talk Dental to avoid trademark issues) and offered advice on whatever was of concern to the patient.

As the patient was present, I could do my own examination and offer an independent opinion, charging $99 for a half hour visit. We usually made use of x-rays from their first-opinion office but took our own if necessary. We did no treatment to make it clear that we had no financial incentive affecting our recommendations.

Our sample of patients is skewed because those who came in were the ones who were suspicious – definitely not a cross-section of all dental patients. But among those patients, my opinion was that almost two-thirds of the recommended work (by dollar value) was unnecessary. I was in agreement with the full treatment recommendation in only one case in twenty.

I also examined the home-care practices of each patient. That individual attention revealed shortcomings that, once corrected, can prevent a host of future problems. People have been very grateful for the service. My estimate that general dentistry costs can be reduced by half comes from this experience.

8. A Final Word

In social settings, the routine question is "What do you do?" When I would say "I'm a dentist", the floodgates would open and personal stories would pour forth. There's the lady who was told she needed four root canals and crowns. She could not afford it and did nothing, yet had no problems in the decades since. There are the people with no problems for years when their aging dentist sells his practice. The new dentist with the half-million dollar practice-purchase loan suddenly "finds" many problems requiring extensive expensive treatment. And there is the frequent tale of how expensive work was recommended on one visit, often with the hard sell, never to be mentioned again in subsequent visits.

Unnecessary treatment is common. It is a major cost that serves only the business needs of the insurer and provider. It is a cost that we can reduce without affecting quality of patient care or its availability.

The practical way to control that excess is to have separate offices providing advice, to make the patient a knowledgeable, empowered consumer. That knowledgeable patient will bring restraint to the unchallenged power of the professionals in the current system.

Three relatively simple changes are necessary: One, empower the patient through private advisory practices that do no treatment. Two, give that patient free rein to shop by eliminating contracted "networks" – they must be able to use their insurance anywhere, just as you would auto insurance. And three, teach prevention in the advisory offices, on an individual level, under a separate billing code to foster wellness. Properly implemented, these three measures have the potential to reduce expenditures for general dentistry by half.

But think beyond dentistry, for these circumstances exist in medicine, law and even government. We are encouraged to trust the professionals, but trust gives them power over us. And power corrupts. You have seen where blind trust can lead in dentistry. The patient or consumer must play a part to avoid exploitation.

George has a local insurance business. I was in his office one day discussing a policy when I explained my work creating a dental advisory service. He struck a thoughtful pose, tilted back in his chair, and considered the idea. "I can see the sense in it," he said. "But it wouldn't apply to me. I've had the same dentist for 17 years, he's a good friend and I love the guy." He wished me well and off I went.

That was in April. Along about September, I get a telephone call and it was George. "I need a second opinion" he said. He came to the office and told me that his dentist wanted to do a crown and take out a wisdom tooth. He really trusted the guy, and didn't want him to know he was checking up on him, but George *really* didn't like the idea of having a tooth pulled. He was hoping I could tell him something different. But in this case, I agreed with his dentist's plan and said the tooth had to go. George was grateful and steeled himself to go back. His trust was warranted, but how is one to know?

Is <u>your</u> work really necessary? How will <u>you</u> know? Trust if you must, but verify.

www.ingramcontent.com/pod-product-compliance
Lightning Source LLC
Chambersburg PA
CBHW050349290526
45785CB00006B/2699